A YEAR
OF
YOU

A YEAR
OF
YOU

A SEASONAL GUIDE TO BOOSTING
YOUR BRILLIANCE

First published in Great Britain 2020 by Trigger

Trigger is a trading style of Shaw Callaghan Ltd & Shaw Callaghan 23 USA, INC.

The Foundation Centre

Navigation House, 48 Millgate, Newark

Nottinghamshire NG24 4TS UK

www.triggerpublishing.com

Text Copyright © 2020 Trigger

British Library Cataloguing in Publication Data

A CIP catalogue record for this book is available upon request
from the British Library

ISBN: 9781789561968

Trigger has asserted its right under the Copyright,
Design and Patents Act 1988 to be identified as the author of this work

Cover design by Bookollective

Typeset by Design Marque

Printed and bound in Great Britain by Clays Ltd, Elcograf S.p.A

How to Use This Book

When life is so busy, it can be hard to find the time to look after yourself. Whether you're studying, working, caring for loved ones or doing your own thing, everyone needs a bit of me-time to achieve a healthy life balance. *A Year of You* can help you do that.

This handy book is jam-packed with prompts, activities, inspirational quotes and pages for reflection, to help you focus on yourself and take back control... as well as pages for you to colour in, which is proven to be a mindful practice.

There's no set way to use this book; you can follow it season by season and week by week, or simply dip in and out whenever you need a boost – it's up to you.

You can add in your own week number at the top of each page, so you can use it as rigidly or as fluidly as you like – to help you get on top of things or to give you some routine.

Turn the page and begin your journey to a better you!

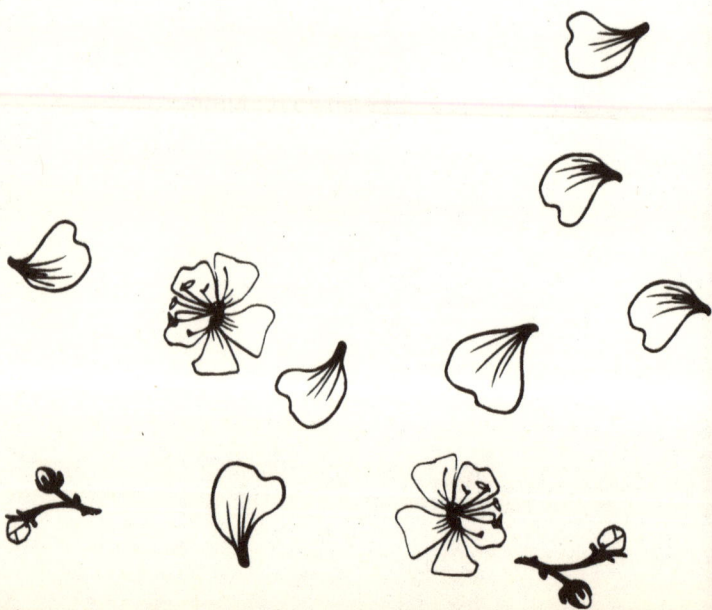

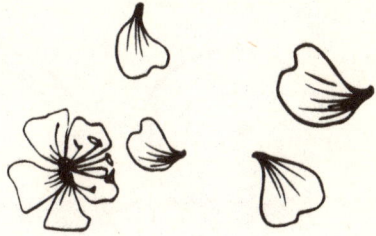

HELLO
Spring

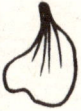

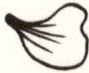

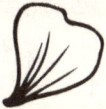

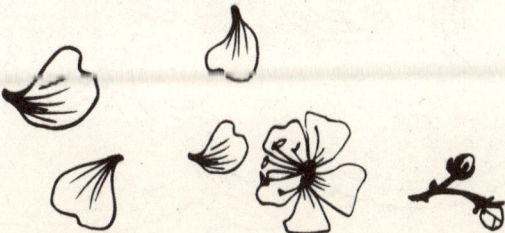

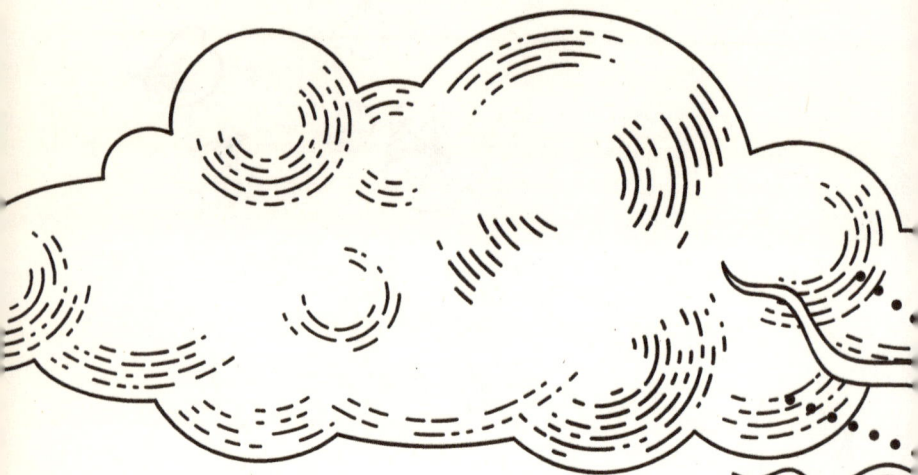

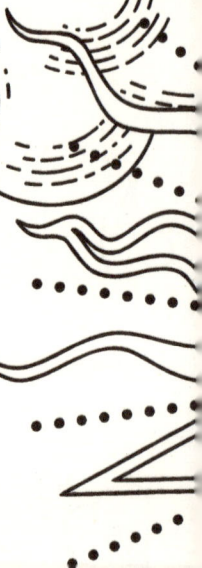

Colour me in as you
mindfully set your
intentions for the
weeks ahead.

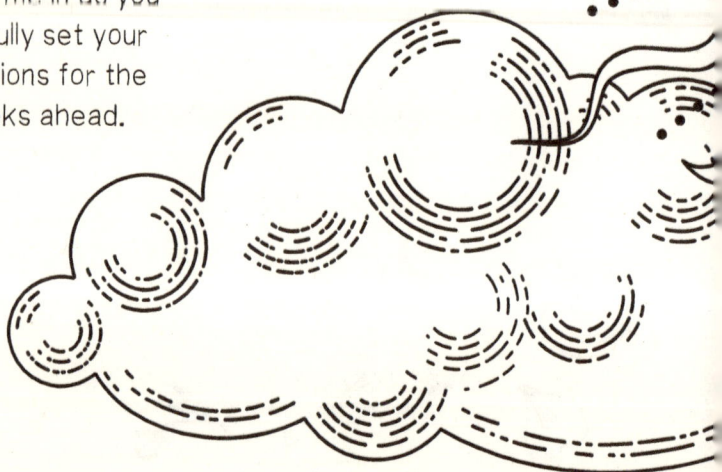

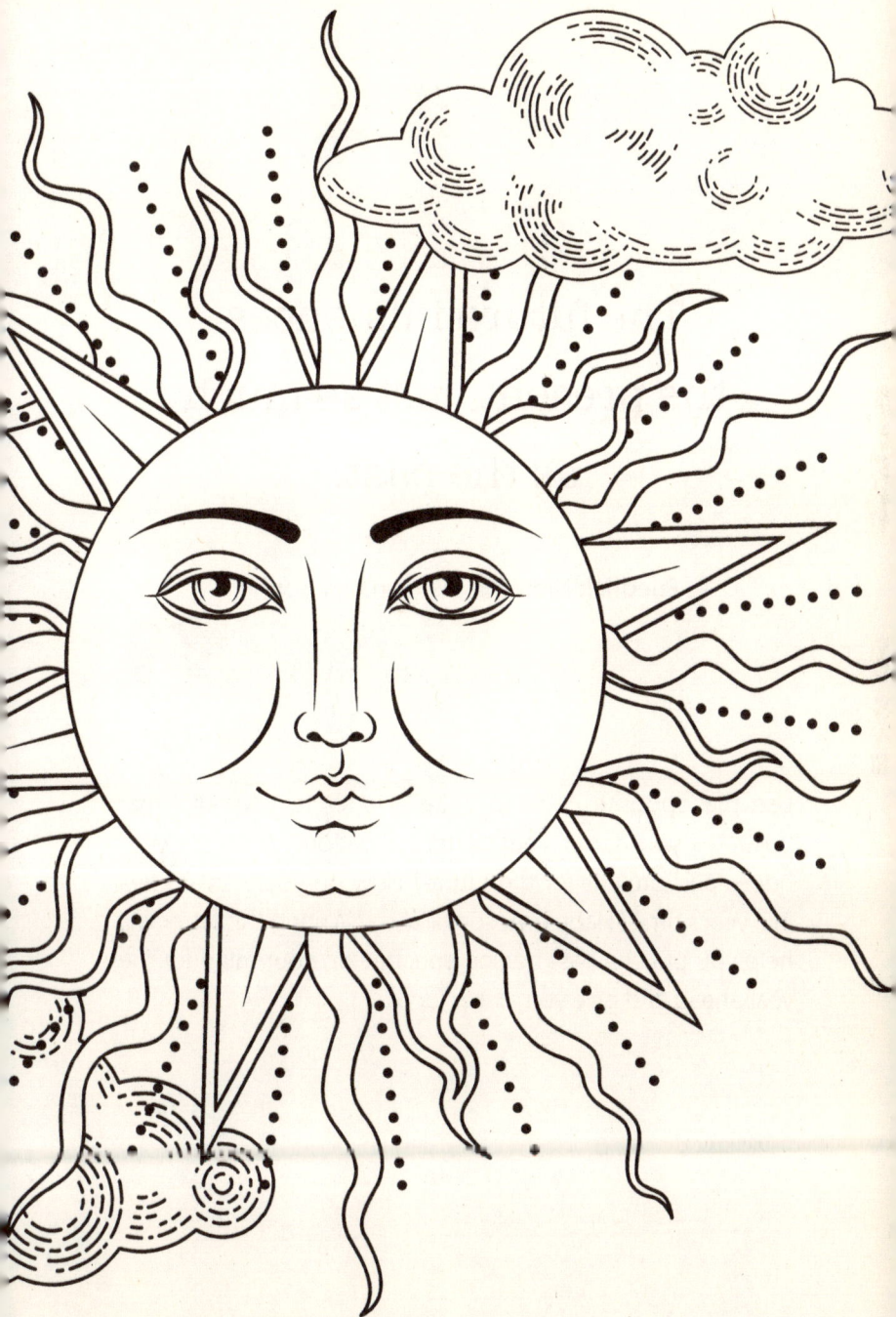

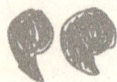

The future influences the present, just as much as the past.

Friedrich Nietzche, German philosopher

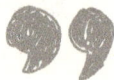

Use the opposite page to write a letter to yourself. What frustrates you about your current situation? What are your hopes and dreams for the future? How do you want to feel in a year's time? Happy? Accomplished? Writing this letter will help you put the past behind you, free up your mind for the year ahead and give you a new focus.

Dear Past Me,

_____

_____

_____

_____

_____

_____

_____

_____

_____

_____

_____

_____

_____

_____

_____

_____

Week _____

_____

_____

_____

_____

_____

_____

_____

_____

_____

_____

_____

_____

_____

_____

_____

_____

Week _____

_____

_____

_____

_____

_____

_____

_____

_____

_____

_____

_____

_____

_____

_____

_____

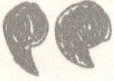

Change the way you look at things, and the things you look at change.

Wayne Dyer, author and motivational speaker

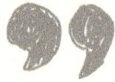

What's on your to-do list this year? To achieve your goals it helps to have a positive mindset, but do you often find that your go-to thoughts are negative? If so, you're not alone. Human beings are hardwired to think cynically by default, but it doesn't have to be that way. How will you inject some positive changes into your life? Use the next page to turn the negative things you tell yourself into something positive. For example, instead of saying "I'm so stupid. Why did I get that wrong?" say "It's human to make mistakes. I'll learn from it."

Week _____

_____

_____

_____

_____

_____

_____

_____

_____

_____

_____

_____

_____

_____

_____

_____

_____

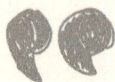

If your compassion does not include yourself, it is incomplete.

Jack Kornfield, author and Buddhist practitioner

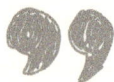

Have you ever made a New Year's resolution that you broke almost immediately? If so, you're not alone. Many of us break our resolutions – and that's because we put a lot of pressure on ourselves to change too much, too soon. Think about the small steps you want to make towards bettering yourself. The key thing here is to make them achievable. Don't end up beating yourself up for not mastering Mandarin in three months! Set yourself goals that have a realistic time frame and write them down.

Week _____

My goals:

_____

_____

_____

_____

_____

_____

_____

_____

_____

_____

_____

_____

_____

_____

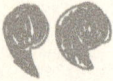

I do find that there's a
fine balance between
preparation and seeing
what happens naturally.

Timothée Chalamet, actor

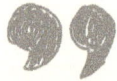

We tend to want to have a hand in everything in life. It makes us feel better if we think we can control what's happening around us. It also makes us stressed when we lose that control. When a situation arises, use the page opposite to assess what, if anything, you can do about it. If you can't do anything, try to let go of that need to be in control, and just relax.

Week _____

_____

_____

_____

_____

_____

_____

_____

_____

_____

_____

_____

_____

_____

_____

_____

_____

_____

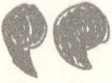

I love who I am.
I love what I've become.

Bernie Mac, comedian and actor

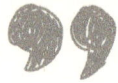

Our minds are so often filled with negative chatter about ourselves. How can you silence this voice and replace it with a more positive one? What do you need to tell yourself more often? Write down some positive affirmations on the page opposite, then read them often. Write all your statements starting with "I" and in the present tense, like in the quote above.

Week _____

_____

_____

_____

_____

_____

_____

_____

_____

_____

_____

_____

_____

_____

_____

_____

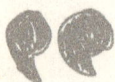

When we refuse to balance the overwhelming demands of work, home, family, friends, and personal growth, stress will be the natural result.

Mary Southerland, author and motivational speaker

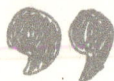

Sometimes life can feel overwhelming. Use the next page to write down what's going on for you at the moment. Is work stressful? Has housework got on top of you? Are you stretching yourself too thin? Take a look at what you've written down and prioritize the areas that are causing you the most stress. Then try to make some changes to find a healthier balance. You'll feel lighter in no time!

Week _____

_____

_____

_____

_____

_____

_____

_____

_____

_____

_____

_____

_____

_____

_____

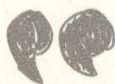

"When you have a bad day, a really bad day, try and

treat the world better than it treated you

Patrick Stump, musician and songwriter

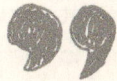

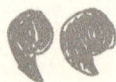

What would life be if we had no courage to attempt anything?

Vincent Van Gogh, painter

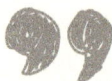

Is there anything you always meant to do but haven't started for some reason – like taking up roller derby or knitting? What's holding you back? We've left some blank pages for you to map out your thoughts and make a plan of action to do what you've always wanted to do. Write whatever comes to mind and don't hold back. Think big! Dream big!

Week _____

My action plan:

_____

_____

_____

_____

_____

_____

_____

_____

_____

_____

_____

_____

_____

_____

_____

_____

Week _____

_____

_____

_____

_____

_____

_____

_____

_____

_____

_____

_____

_____

_____

_____

_____

_____

Week ____

_____

_____

_____

_____

_____

_____

_____

_____

_____

_____

_____

_____

_____

_____

_____

_____

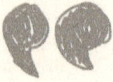

Clutter is nothing more than postponed decisions.

Barbara Hemphill, professional organizer

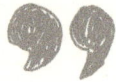

With the widespread adoption of Scandinavian wellbeing terms such as *hygge*, *lagom* and *lykke*, spring cleaning is a year-round trend, but the emergence of spring is as good a reason as any to tackle those bulging cupboards and drawers. As well as giving you a more relaxed and streamlined living space, decluttering is such a mindful and relaxing practice. Get rid of that faded sweater that you don't even wear to hang around the house in anymore, and donate those mugs that you hate. Surround yourself with stuff you love, and space to breathe.

Get started by making three piles:

1. Bin

2. Recycle/resell

3. Donate

Keep these tips in mind as you sort:

* Don't try to clear your whole house at once. Split the task into rooms or even segments of time, that way you'll avoid tidying-induced burnout!

* Thrift shops generally sell clothes that look new or nearly new. If something doesn't fit into that category, reconsider what to do with it. If any of your possessions are no longer fit for purpose and can't be mended or sold on, stick them on the throw-away pile.

* Struggling to decide what to keep? If you haven't worn it or used it for a year, you probably don't want it. That said, don't throw everything out in a frenzy; if you really are hesitating over something, keep hold of it for now. This is an ongoing exercise; you don't need to finish it all in one day – and you definitely don't want to regret getting rid of something!

* If an item is of sentimental value to you, keep it.

* With the resurgence of upcycling, there are lots of Facebook groups and online communities you can join to get more ideas about reusing, repurposing and repairing your things.

Use the pages overleaf to note any feelings that come up from releasing yourself of unwanted possessions.

_____

_____

_____

_____

_____

_____

_____

_____

_____

_____

_____

_____

_____

_____

_____

_____

Week _____

_____

_____

_____

_____

_____

_____

_____

_____

_____

_____

_____

_____

_____

_____

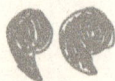

In the spring, at the end of the day, you should smell like dirt.

Margaret Atwood, poet and author

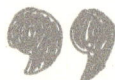

It's amazing what a bit of greenery can do for your spirits. This week, get a plant, and watch it grow. Keep it alive through all the hardships it faces – your partner overwatering it, your cat eating it – and connect with nature.

Colour in the page opposite for a dose of mindfulness.

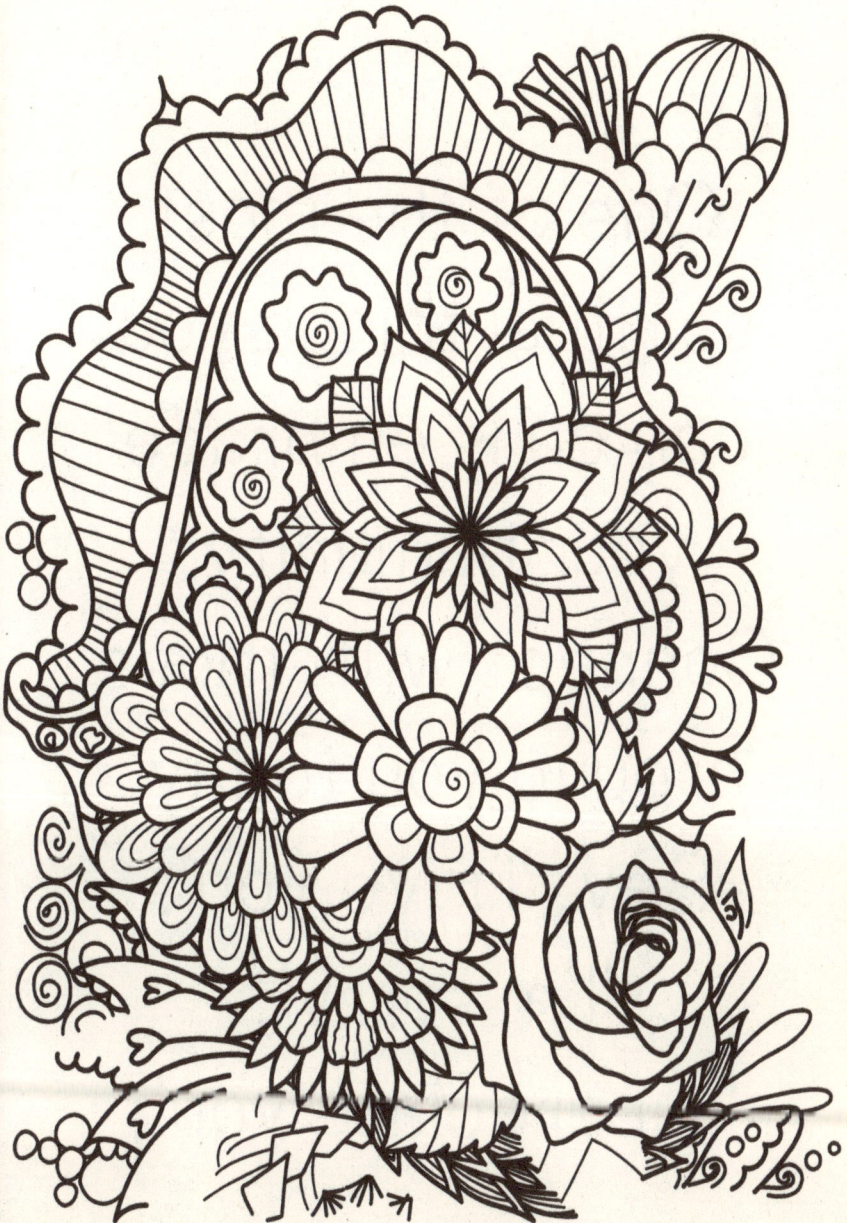

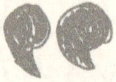

One of the most spiritual things you can do is embrace your humanity. Connect with those around you today. Say, 'I love you', 'I'm sorry', 'I appreciate you',

'I'm proud of you'...
whatever you're
feeling.
Send random
texts, write a cute
note, embrace your
truth and share it ...

Steve Maraboli, author and motivational speaker

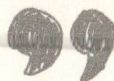

Who haven't you connected with in a while? Write down a list of things you'd like to do for loved ones, and pledge to do one a day for the next little while.

My pledge to loved ones:

1. _____

2. _____

3. _____

4. _____

5. _____

6. _____

7. _____

8. _____

9. _____

10. _____

Week _____

_____

_____

_____

_____

_____

_____

_____

_____

_____

_____

_____

_____

_____

_____

_____

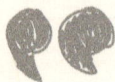

If one cannot enjoy reading a book over and over again, there is no use in reading it at all.

Oscar Wilde, poet and playwright

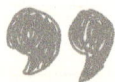

Books can contain so much more than the words on the page. Grab a book off your shelf, close your eyes and point to a sentence at random. What is it? What do you think when you see it? Write it down and see what ideas it sparks. You might even discover something new about yourself!

Week ____

_____

_____

_____

_____

_____

_____

_____

_____

_____

_____

_____

_____

_____

_____

_____

_____

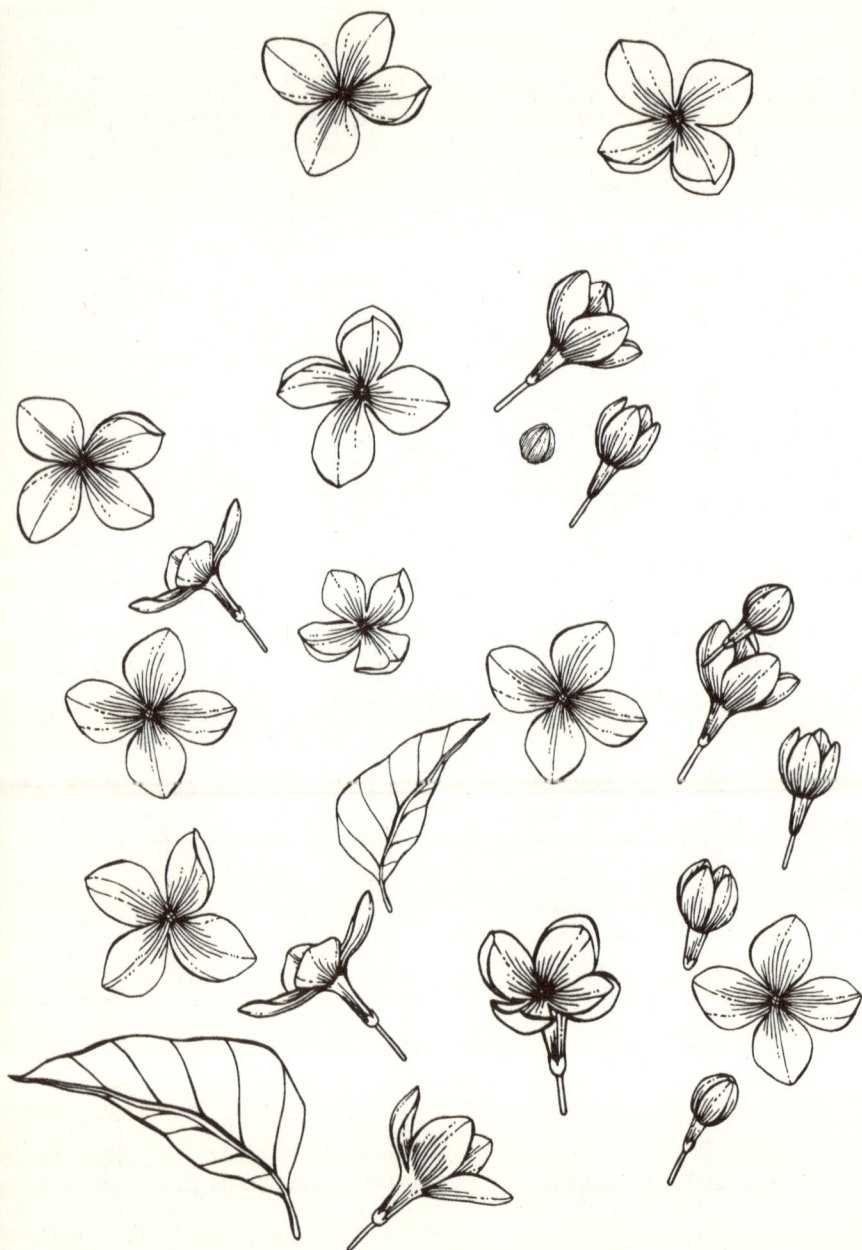

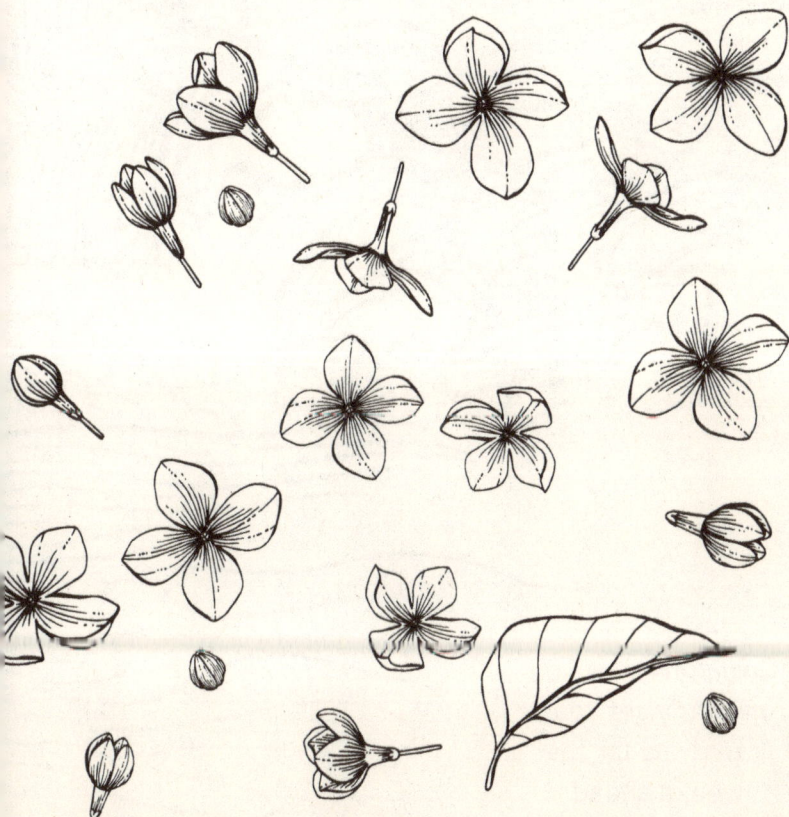

HELLO
Summer

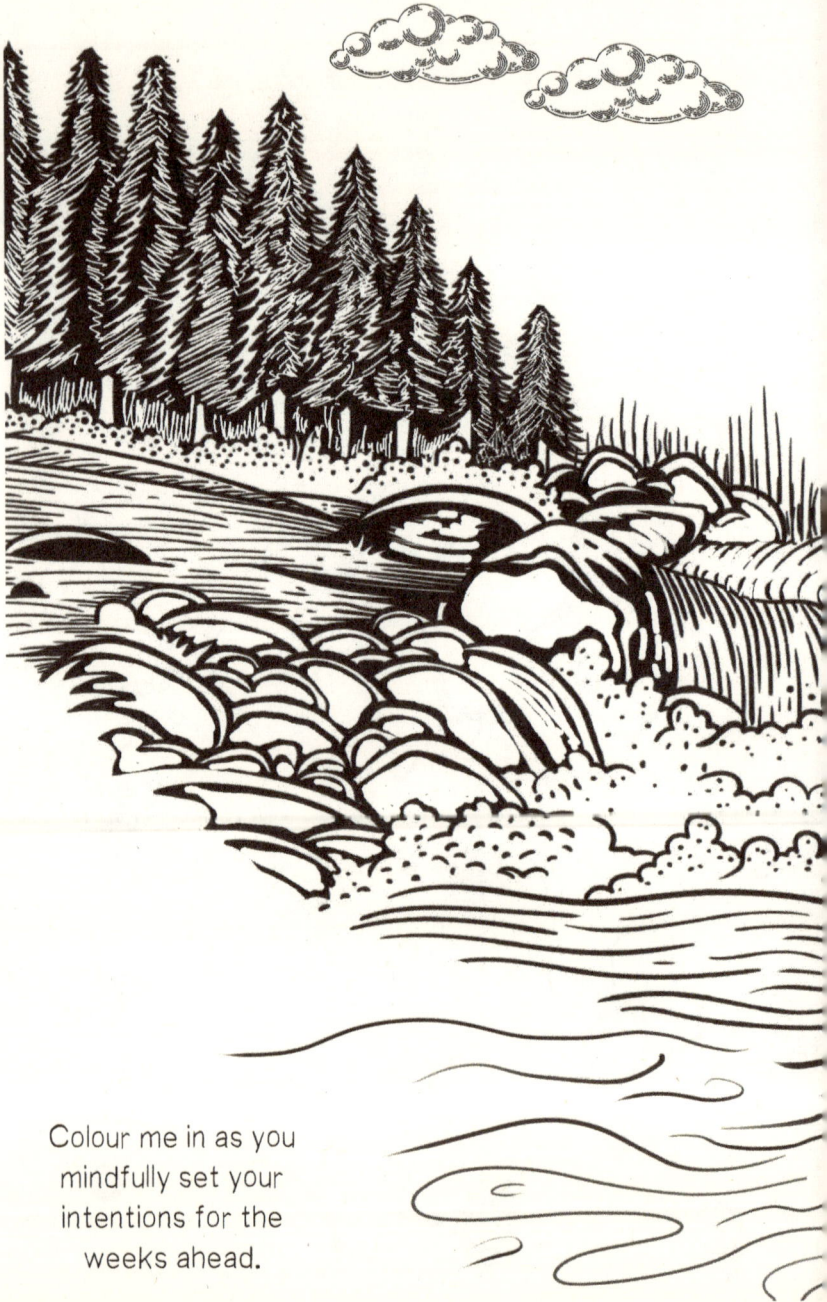

Colour me in as you
mindfully set your
intentions for the
weeks ahead.

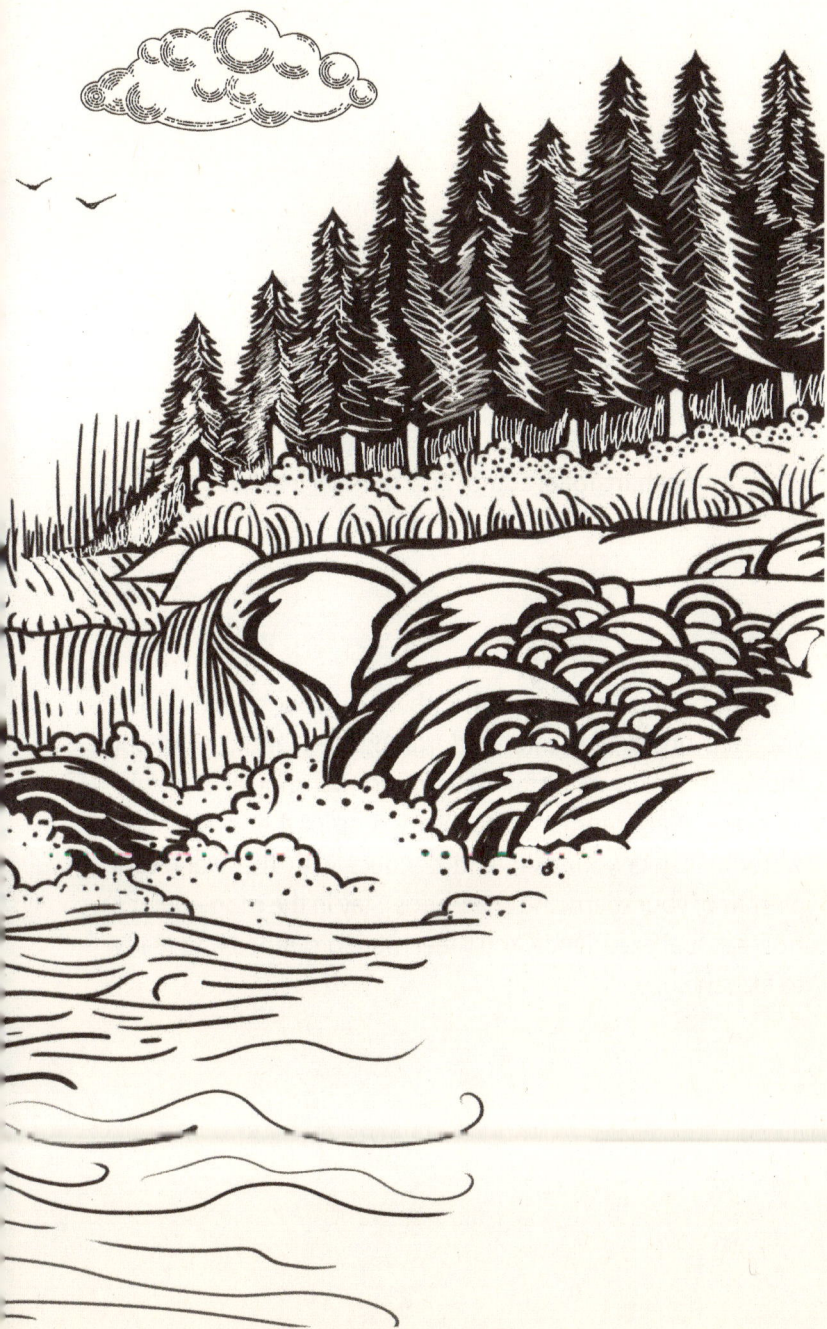

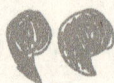

Wherever you are, be there totally.

Eckhart Tolle, author and spiritual teacher

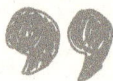

Is having a shower just another thing on your to-do list? Do you step under the water and immediately get lost in your thoughts? This week, stay mindful as you shower and fully embrace every moment. Feel every drop of the invigorating water as it hits your skin, and connect with the wonderful aromas of your soaps and shampoos. Stay in the moment for a truly sensual experience. You'll feel more grounded and ready to face the day.

Week _____

_____

_____

_____

_____

_____

_____

_____

_____

_____

_____

_____

_____

_____

_____

_____

_____

_____

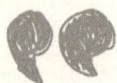

> Spend less time tearing yourself apart, worrying if you're good enough. You are good enough.

Reese Witherspoon, actress

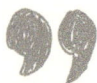

Get into the habit of writing your worries down and tackling them one by one (there's a space opposite to get you started). This way, you'll be able to see them for what they are and work through them. You might find they're not as big a deal as you thought!

Week _____

My worries:

_____

_____

_____

_____

_____

_____

_____

_____

_____

_____

_____

_____

_____

_____

_____

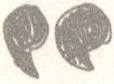

Listen to silence.
It has so much to say.

Rumi, poet

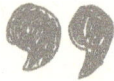

We are often surrounded by so much noise that silence can feel uncomfortable, not least because it leaves us alone with our own thoughts. This week, take out those headphones while you're walking, turn off the radio or TV while you're eating – you just might find it cathartic to make some quiet time for "just being". Reflect on how it felt for you.

Week _____

_____

_____

_____

_____

_____

_____

_____

_____

_____

_____

_____

_____

_____

_____

_____

_____

_____

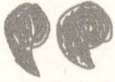

Summer afternoon — summer afternoon; to me those have always been the two most beautiful words in the English language.

Henry James, author

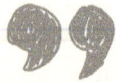

Week _____

_____

_____

_____

_____

_____

_____

_____

_____

_____

_____

_____

_____

_____

_____

_____

Week _____

_____

_____

_____

_____

_____

_____

_____

_____

_____

_____

_____

_____

_____

_____

_____

_____

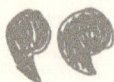

Life is like riding a bicycle. To keep your balance, you must keep moving.

Albert Einstein, physicist

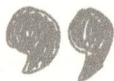

Making changes is hard, but so worth it. It might take time, but keep going! Keep in mind the definition of perseverance – "continued effort to do or achieve something despite difficulties, failure, or opposition." (Merriam Webster). Use the next page to remind yourself why you're on this journey. Reflect again on what it is you're trying to achieve.

Week _____

_____

_____

_____

_____

_____

_____

_____

_____

_____

_____

_____

_____

_____

_____

_____

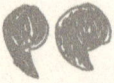

"I don't have to take a trip around the world or be on a yacht in the Mediterranean to have happiness.

I can find it in the little things, like looking out into my backyard and seeing deer in the fields.

Queen Latifah,
rapper, singer songwriter, actor and producer

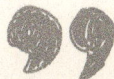

Week _____

_____

_____

_____

_____

_____

_____

_____

_____

_____

_____

_____

_____

_____

_____

Week _____

_____

_____

_____

_____

_____

_____

_____

_____

_____

_____

_____

_____

_____

_____

_____

_____

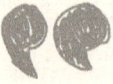

> Carry out a random act
> of kindness, with no
> expectation of reward,
> safe in the knowledge that
> one day someone might
> do the same for you.

Diana, Princess of Wales

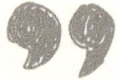

What do you consider to be random acts of kindness? Helping an elderly person across the road? Making your colleague a cup of tea when they're stressed? Tipping someone a bit more than usual? What have you done lately to make someone's day?

Week _____

_____

_____

_____

_____

_____

_____

_____

_____

_____

_____

_____

_____

_____

_____

_____

_____

_____

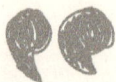

You have to stop crying, and you have to go kick some ass.

Lady Gaga, singer-songwriter

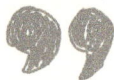

If life's been a bit tough lately – or even if it hasn't – stop for a moment. Make a list on the opposite page of reasons you're awesome, and read them aloud to yourself. Remember, you've got this!

Week _____

Reasons I am awesome:

_____

_____

_____

_____

_____

_____

_____

_____

_____

_____

_____

_____

_____

_____

_____

_____

_____

_____

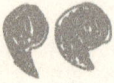

You can live the
life you want.
And that life
can be amazing.

Hope Virgo, author and mental health campaigner

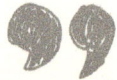

Week ____

_____

_____

_____

_____

_____

_____

_____

_____

_____

_____

_____

_____

_____

_____

_____

_____

_____

_____

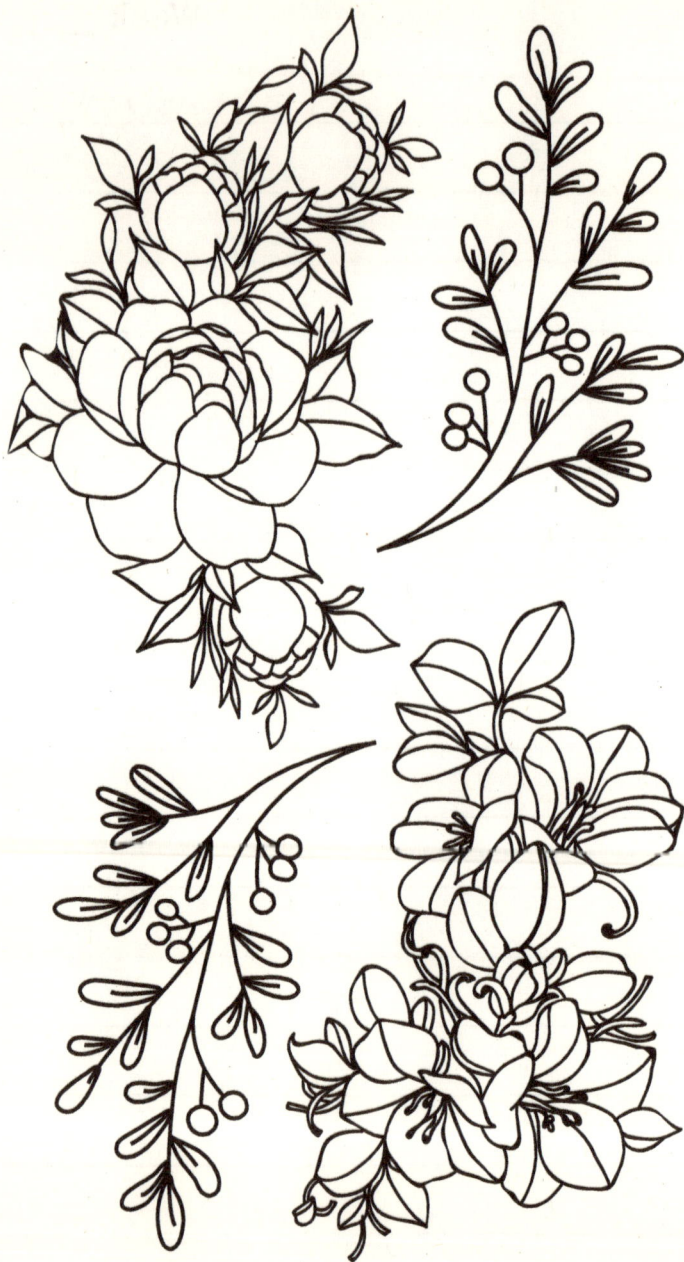

Week _____

_____

_____

_____

_____

_____

_____

_____

_____

_____

_____

_____

_____

_____

_____

_____

_____

_____

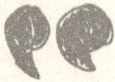

Take rest; a field that
has rested gives a
bountiful crop.

Ovid, poet

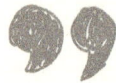

When life is busy, it's easy to put yourself at the bottom of your to-do list. This week, take a moment to do something just for you. Plan your actions on the self-care action plan page overleaf. Here are a few ideas to get you started…

Mood Music
Do you need to get psyched up? Make an upbeat playlist. Need a mental health day? Stream calming songs and ride it out. Miss being on holiday? Pick summery tunes, world music, or songs that remind you of past holidays.

Write It Out
Take up a pen (or use a notes app on your phone) and start writing. Escape into another world for a little while. You don't have to write a novel; even free verse can be cathartic.

Lose Yourself in a Book or a Movie
Dive into another world to escape for a bit. It's mindfulness with minimal effort, and a treat for the senses.

Bake it Off
Try creating something delicious as a distraction. It will keep your mind busy, your hands full, and your tummy happy. Plus it makes the house smell divine, and is a great excuse to connect with loved ones. Cookie, anyone?

Phone a Friend
If you're feeling rubbish, don't be afraid to reach out to someone. After all, that's what friends are for.

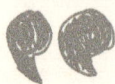

Shall I compare thee to a summer's day? Thou art more lovely and more temperate.

William Shakespeare, playwright

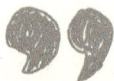

My self-care action plan:

_____

_____

_____

_____

_____

_____

_____

_____

_____

_____

_____

_____

_____

_____

_____

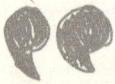

Live the actual moment. Only this actual moment is life. Don't be attached to the future. Don't worry about things ...

Don't think about getting up or taking off to do anything. Don't think about 'departing.'

Thich Nhat Hanh,
Buddhist monk and peace activist

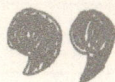

Week _____

_____

_____

_____

_____

_____

_____

_____

_____

_____

_____

_____

_____

_____

_____

_____

_____

_____

HELLO

Autumn

Colour me in as you
mindfully set your
intentions for the
weeks ahead.

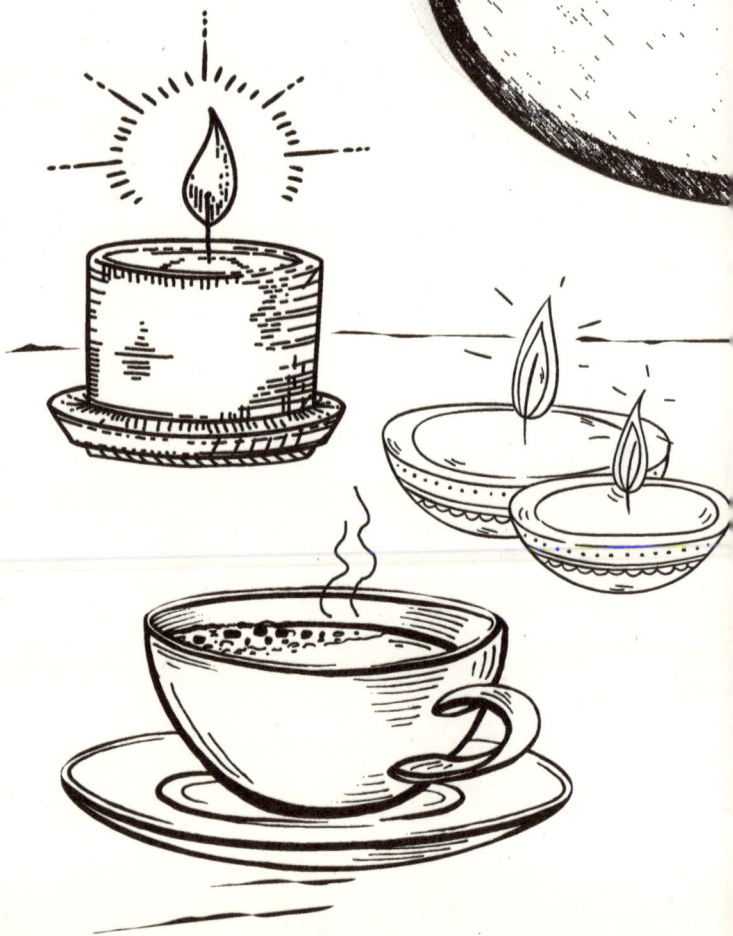

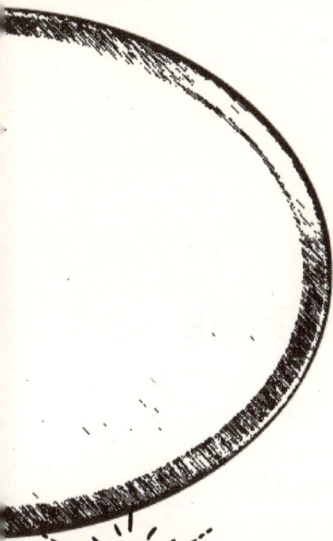

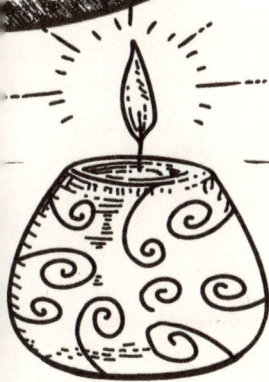

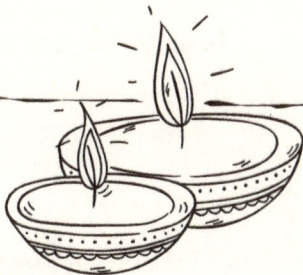

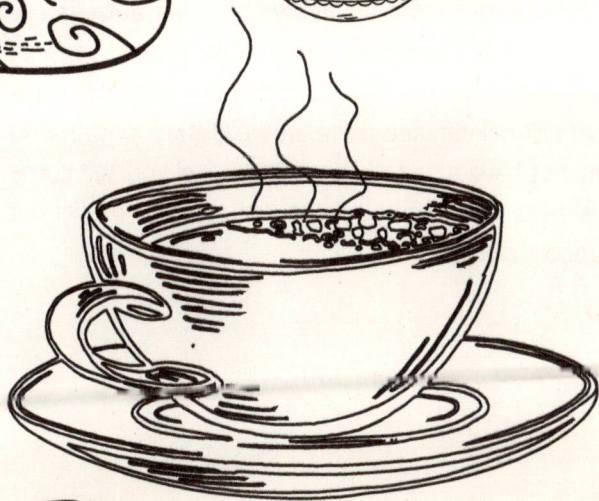

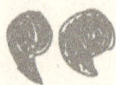

You're only given a little spark of madness. You mustn't lose it.

Robin Williams, actor

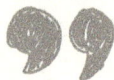

There's a technique known as "freewriting" that authors use to get their creative juices flowing. In its most basic sense, it involves the person writing freely and without thought about anything at all, making sure there are no distractions around them. Why not have a go? Write until you feel yourself come to a natural stop – you might be surprised at what you get out of your subconscious!

Week _____

_____

_____

_____

_____

_____

_____

_____

_____

_____

_____

_____

_____

_____

_____

_____

_____

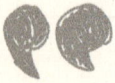

Does saying 'I am standard'
make me average?
Absolutely not.
I just meet new standards
that I now understand
are the real ones.

Lucy Nichol, writer and mental health campaigner

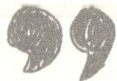

Through writing in this book, what realizations have you come
to about who you are and what your goals are for the future?

Week _____

My goals and realizations:

_____

_____

_____

_____

_____

_____

_____

_____

_____

_____

_____

_____

_____

_____

_____

_____

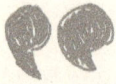

How often do you carve out space for yourself? When in your day can you stop and really pay attention to what is going on for you?

How recently have you stopped to consider your hopes and dreams?

Gemma Cribb, clinical psychologist

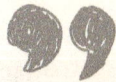

"

Way too many people feel like they can only like themselves if they change. Here are self-love expert Gemma Cribb's top five tips for a new way of viewing yourself:

1. Write an inventory of what you are proud of having done. We are often so focused on what we haven't achieved that we forget to recognize what we have!

2. Make a list of all the people who have made positive contributions, no matter how small, to your life and resolve to thank them. Changing your focus to gratitude and abundance will not only lift your mood, it will attract more people to you as well!

3. Ask your best friend or a close family member to tell you what they really appreciate or admire about you.

4. Imagine you were an "honored guest" in your house. How would you make a guest feel welcome and cared for? Would you cook special food? Clean up the house? Buy fresh flowers? Pick your favourite of these things and resolve to do this for yourself regularly, whether you feel you deserve it or not. You are worthy of love and care, no matter what.

5. Think of one thing that you do, or one aspect of yourself, that you find difficult to like or approve of. Tune in to when you are having negative thoughts about this behaviour and instead of berating yourself yet again, resolve to turn towards yourself with compassion. Thinking "Awww poor thing, it's okay, I'm here for you," is far more powerful than criticism, and you'll be surprised at how it changes seemingly stuck patterns!

Week _____

_____

_____

_____

_____

_____

_____

_____

_____

_____

_____

_____

_____

_____

_____

_____

_____

_____

_____

_____

_____

_____

_____

_____

_____

_____

_____

_____

_____

_____

_____

_____

Week _____

_____

_____

_____

_____

_____

_____

_____

_____

_____

_____

_____

_____

_____

_____

_____

_____

_____

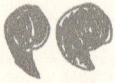

We ourselves feel that
we are a drop in the
ocean. But the ocean
would be less because
of that missing drop.

Mother Teresa, Roman Catholic nun and missionary

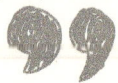

Week _____

_____

_____

_____

_____

_____

_____

_____

_____

_____

_____

_____

_____

_____

_____

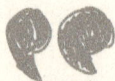

Everything is about balance. You can't work, work, work, work without any play.

Janelle Monáe, singer-songwriter, actor and producer

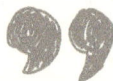

We all get into a solid routine but sometimes, the weeks can feel monotonous, and weekend breaks always go too quickly. This seemingly never-ending cycle can cause low moods and bring you down, especially when you feel like you never leave your desk! So, why not shake things up a bit?

Plan a weekend of fun, whether with your friends, family or partner. Go white water rafting, climbing, or even just take a weekend to explore a new city. Add a bit of fun and spontaneity to your life, and break out of that rut. Write down your ideas.

Week _____

My big weekend:

_____

_____

_____

_____

_____

_____

_____

_____

_____

_____

_____

_____

_____

_____

_____

_____

_____

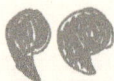

Whether you come from a council estate or a country estate, your success will be determined by your own confidence and fortitude.

Michelle Obama, author, lawyer and former First Lady

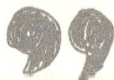

What are you the proudest of in your life? List your best achievements, big or small, on the next page.

Week _____

My achievements:

_____

_____

_____

_____

_____

_____

_____

_____

_____

_____

_____

_____

_____

_____

_____

_____

Week _____

_____

_____

_____

_____

_____

_____

_____

_____

_____

_____

_____

_____

_____

_____

_____

_____

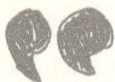

> I can recall all the snakes
> that tried to bite me,
> but I prefer to think of all
> those who dared me to dream
> by offering me a step up.

Pete Roberts, author

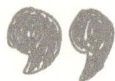

Who are you thankful to for making you who you are? Perhaps it's a teacher, an old school friend, a grandparent... Use the next page to reflect on who's on your list and what they did to help you, and then tell them or write them a letter. If they are no longer part of your life, still express your thoughts in writing – you will find yourself lighter for doing so, and it's fulfilling to boot.

Week _____

_____

_____

_____

_____

_____

_____

_____

_____

_____

_____

_____

_____

_____

_____

_____

_____

_____

_____

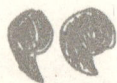

Believing that you are enough is what gives you the courage to be authentic.

Brené Brown, research professor and author

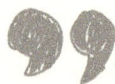

We often strive for perfection when that's simply unattainable. Instead, appreciate yourself for who you are. Look in the mirror and tell yourself, "I am enough." Stick a reminder up if you need to!

Colour in the reminders on the next two pages, then copy them onto sticky notes and leave them where you will see them regularly, as little positive affirmations.

"I am more than
enough just
as I am."

"I am more than
enough just
as I am."

"I am more than
enough just
as I am."

"I am more than
enough just
as I am."

"I am more than
enough just
as I am."

"I am more than
enough just
as I am."

Week _____

_____

_____

_____

_____

_____

_____

_____

_____

_____

_____

_____

_____

_____

_____

_____

_____

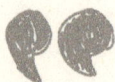

Dreams are illustrations... from the book your soul is writing about you.

Marsha Norman, playwright and novelist

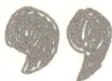

This week, note down your dreams. Use them to initiate creativity, and draw or write a scene based on them. What do you think they're trying to tell you? Keep a notebook by your bed to record your dreams when you wake up, and reflect on them.

Week _____

_____

_____

_____

_____

_____

_____

_____

_____

_____

_____

_____

_____

_____

_____

_____

_____

_____

Week _____

“

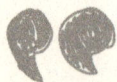

To be nobody but yourself in a world that's doing its best to make you somebody else, is to fight

the hardest
battle you are ever
going to fight.
Never stop
fighting.

E.E. Cummings, poet

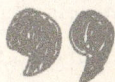

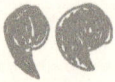

When life puts you in tough situations, don't say, 'Why me?' Just say, 'Try me'.

Dwayne "The Rock" Johnson, actor and former wrestler

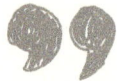

Sometimes we get so bogged down by life's challenges that we forget to celebrate our achievements in overcoming them. This week, take some time to think about all the tough times that you've come through even when you thought you couldn't.

Week _____

_____

_____

_____

_____

_____

_____

_____

_____

_____

_____

_____

_____

_____

_____

_____

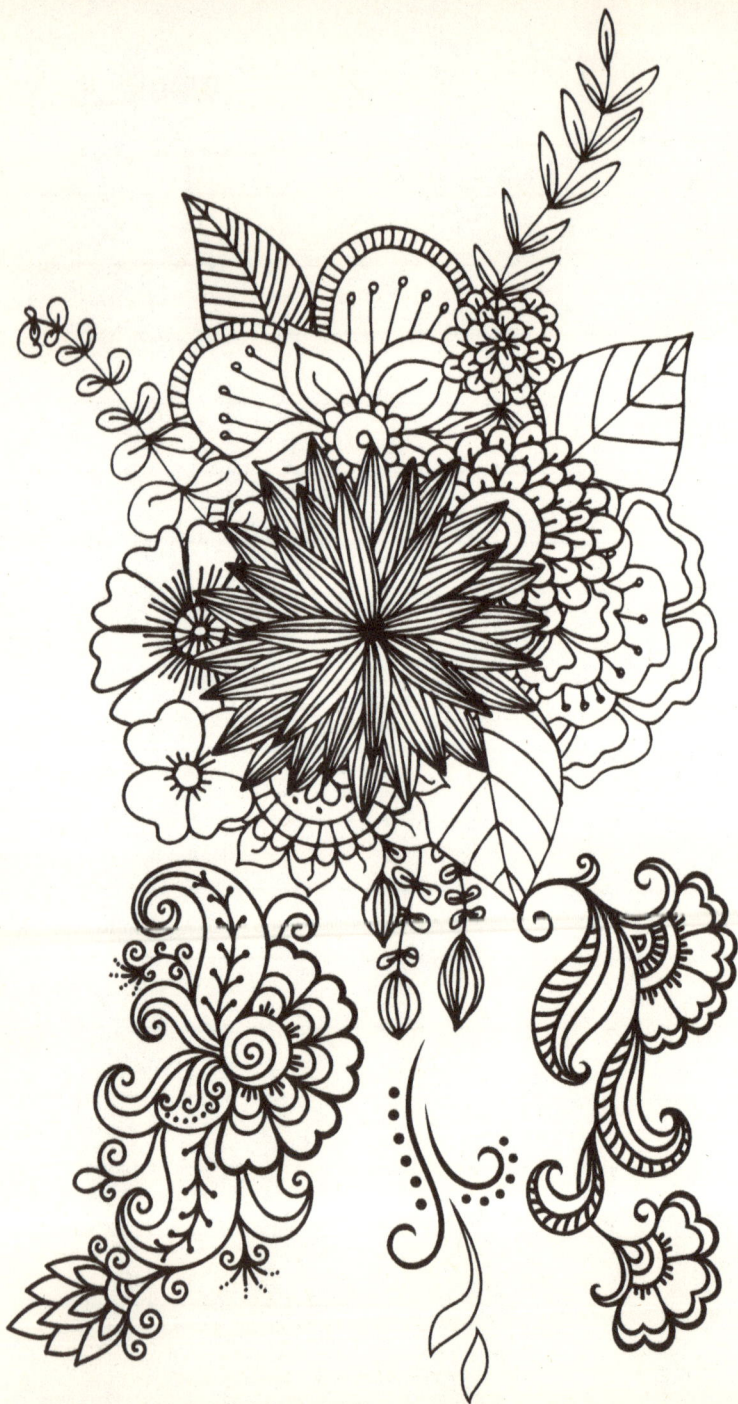

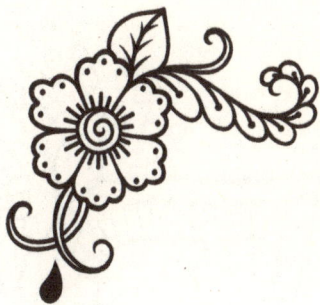
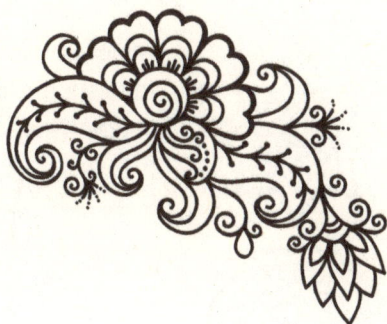

HELLO

Winter

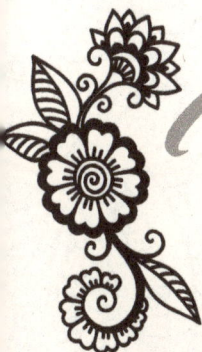
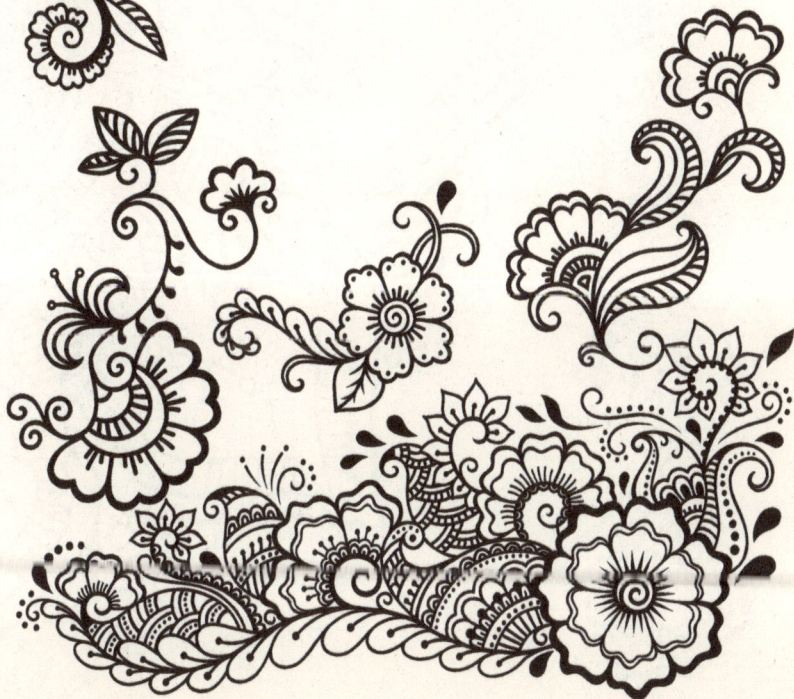

Colour me in as you mindfully set your intentions for the weeks ahead.

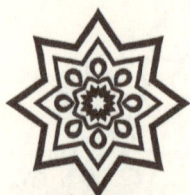

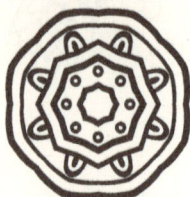

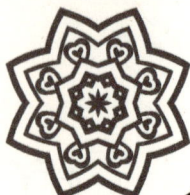

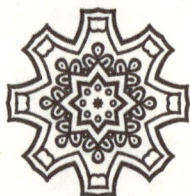

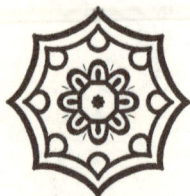

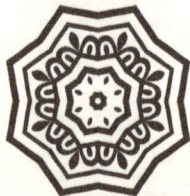

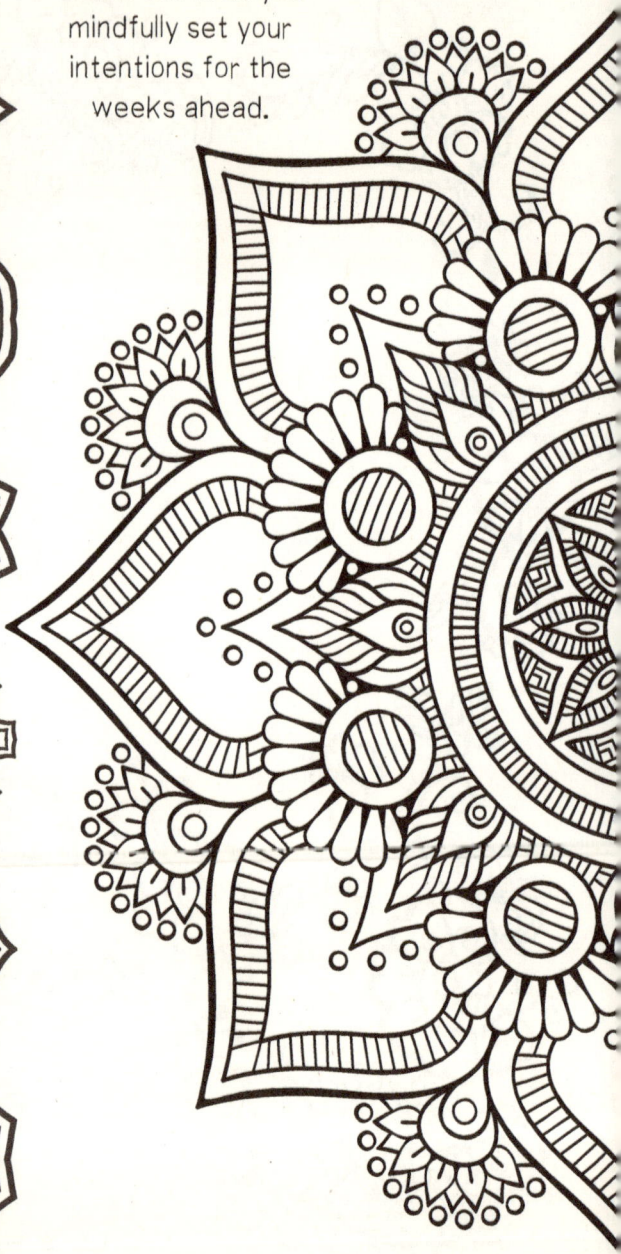

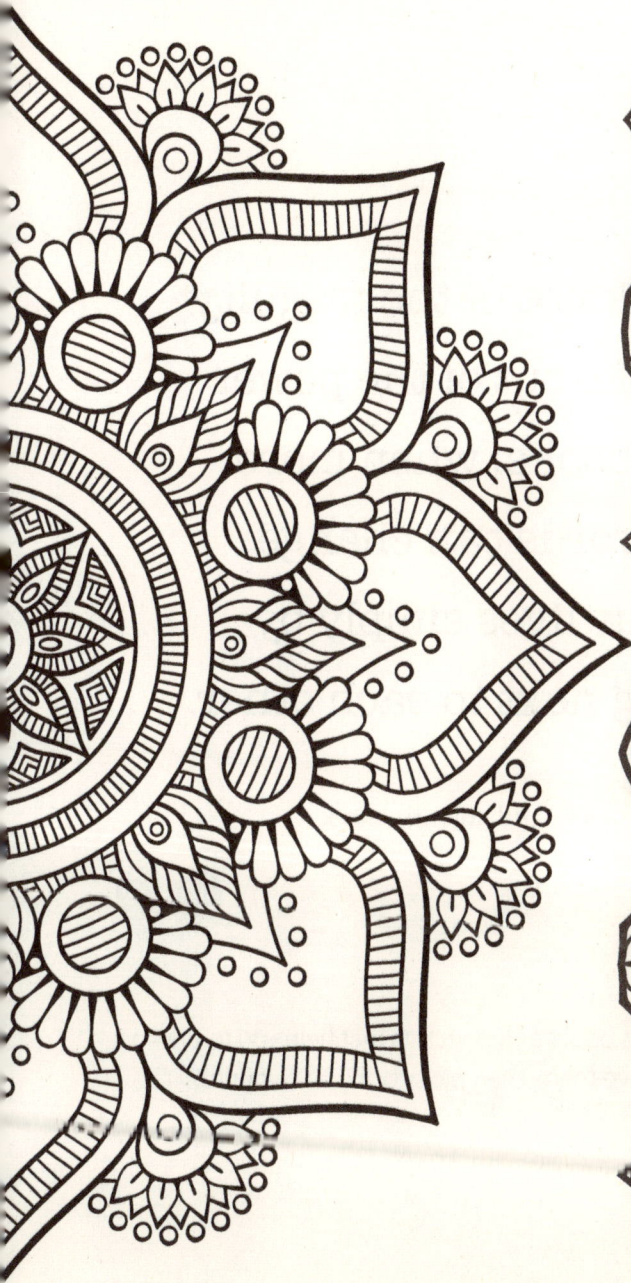

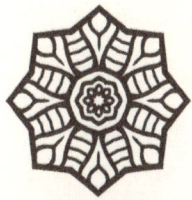

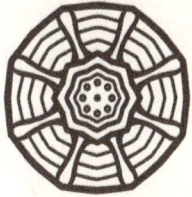

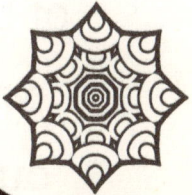

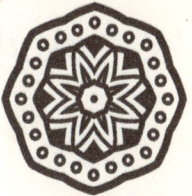

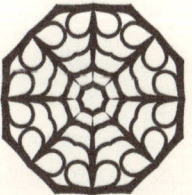

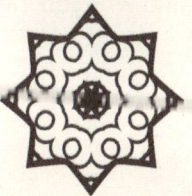

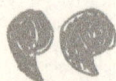

> Think not of the fragility
> of life, but of the power
> of books, when mere
> words can change
> our lives simply by
> being next to each other.

Kamand Kojouri, author

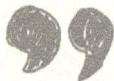

List your top ten books and podcasts that help you to unwind, and why you love them, then pick up an old favourite!

My Top Ten Books/Podcasts:

1. _____

2. _____

3. _____

4. _____

5. _____

6. _____

7. _____

8. _____

9. _____

10. _____

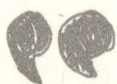

" Your need for acceptance can make you invisible in this world. Don't let anything stand in the way of the light

that shines
through this form.
Risk being seen
in all of
your glory.

Jim Carrey, author

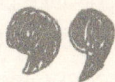

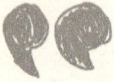

> We don't stop playing
> because we grow old;
> we grow old because
> we stop playing.

George Bernard Shaw, playwright

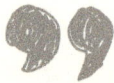

It's important to reconnect with your 'inner child' — the childlike part of you — every so often. It helps you take your mind off the pressures of being a grown-up, and helps to renew and add colour to your world so that you can tackle problems from a different perspective afterwards. Over the page are some ways to be playful, have a good laugh, relax, and de-stress.

Week _____

_____

_____

_____

_____

_____

_____

_____

_____

_____

_____

_____

_____

_____

_____

_____

_____

Talk to your Pet

Just sharing your worries can make you feel better, even if you don't feel ready to talk to a loved one just yet.

Pets are great listeners, too. When you take the dog for a walk first thing in the morning, or clean out your rabbit's hutch, why not unburden your worries and see how they respond. Often, pets will react to how you're feeling, from cues they take from your tone of voice.

Daydream

It might sound easy, but many of us find it hard to let our minds drift because they are stuffed with to-do lists.

Daydreaming has been proven to work wonders for de-stressing and is, in fact, an essential ingredient in creativity and innovation. Set yourself a timer for one minute to start with (or three if you're feeling it), then look out of the window. Find something of interest – maybe a leaf in the wind, maybe a runner, or a little bird – and watch it, follow it, ask yourself where it may be going, or how it may be feeling today … and let your imagination roam.

You might dream about what life will be like ten years down the road, or you might simply be mesmerized by the leaf floating in the air. There is no right or wrong. Just let your mind wander…

Dance

Upbeat music is an instant mood-lifter, and helps you to lose yourself in the moment. Not only that, but dancing is really great exercise and gets your heart rate up. Our instinct as humans is to move to rhythm, so stick on your favourite playlist, and see where the rhythm takes you!

Week _____

_____

_____

_____

_____

_____

_____

_____

_____

_____

_____

_____

_____

_____

_____

_____

_____

Week _____

_____

_____

_____

_____

_____

_____

_____

_____

_____

_____

_____

_____

_____

_____

_____

_____

_____

Week _____

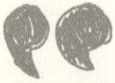

Bathing is my hobby. I do have a hand-carved tub out of marble and onyx ... it was carved to the shape of my body. I told you ... I'm serious about it.

Oprah Winfrey, media executive and talk show host

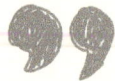

Take some time to pamper and really indulge yourself. Run a deep bath. Throw in a bath bomb, or even some essential oils or fresh flowers. Make it a treat for your senses and imagine your stresses washing away down the drain ...

Week _____

_____

_____

_____

_____

_____

_____

_____

_____

_____

_____

_____

_____

_____

_____

_____

_____

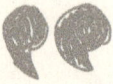

"No one can make you feel inferior without your consent."

Eleanor Roosevelt, activist and former First Lady

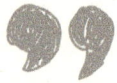

Using gadgets is part of everyday life, but so often they leave us feeling drained and lacking. Take a look at your relationship with technology. How healthy is it? Are you constantly checking social media? Do the posts you read often leave you feeling worse rather than better? Do you feel anxious if you can't find your phone or if the battery is low? Use the page opposite to reflect and then experiment with making small changes, such as limiting your time on social media and having a digital detox, especially when you're with loved ones, at mealtimes and before bedtime. When you've tried it a few times, reflect again on how it felt.

Week _____

_____

_____

_____

_____

_____

_____

_____

_____

_____

_____

_____

_____

_____

_____

_____

_____

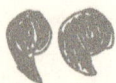

The gem cannot be polished without friction, nor man perfected without trials.

Chinese Proverb

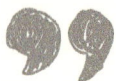

Week ____

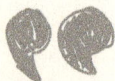

We think we listen, but very rarely do we listen with real understanding, true empathy.

Carl Rogers, humanistic psychologist

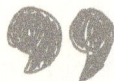

When did you last properly listen? Often, we switch off during conversations or interrupt to tell our own story. This week, take the time to actively listen to your friends, your partner, your children. Make eye contact, focus on their non-verbal communication, such as body language and facial expressions, as well as what they're saying. Reflect on the page opposite about how it felt to be fully present and to truly connect with someone.

Week _____

_____

_____

_____

_____

_____

_____

_____

_____

_____

_____

_____

_____

_____

_____

_____

_____

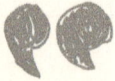

It's how you cope with the bad stuff, both big and little, the nature of your relationship with it, and the attitude you adopt when dealing with it. That's what counts.

Mark Simmonds, author

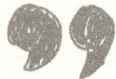

Week _____

_____

_____

_____

_____

_____

_____

_____

_____

_____

_____

_____

_____

_____

_____

_____

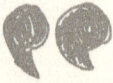

You yourself, as much as anybody in the entire universe, deserve your love and affection.

Sharon Salzberg, author and Buddhist teacher

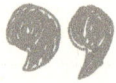

Take the time to practise this simple self-kindness exercise. Sit in a position that feels comfortable and place one hand over your heart, then repeat phrases such as "May I be content", "May I be fulfilled", "May I be healthy". Choose whichever phrases resonate with you. If you find self-compassion difficult to begin with, first practise by imagining saying the phrases to someone you love, such as "May you be content," etc., and then, over time, direct the phrases towards yourself.

Week _____

_____

_____

_____

_____

_____

_____

_____

_____

_____

_____

_____

_____

_____

_____

_____

_____

_____

_____

_____

_____

_____

_____

_____

_____

_____

_____

_____

_____

_____

_____

_____

_____

_____

_____

Week _____

"

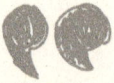

People often say
that they deal
with whatever life
throws at them,
and while that's
okay for those
people, it's not how

I choose to live my life now.
I do the opposite
— I throw myself
at life and let it deal
with me.

Adam Shaw, author and philanthropist

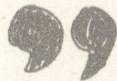

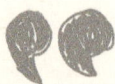

I used to think that confidence came from what other people thought about me but now I realise it comes from what I feel about myself.

Demi Lovato, singer-songwriter

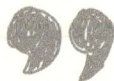

Take the time to reflect on the last year. Write another letter about your current situation. What are your hopes, dreams, wishes, regrets? Compare this letter with the one you wrote in Week 1. What has changed?

Week _____

A letter to myself...

_____

_____

_____

_____

_____

_____

_____

_____

_____

_____

_____

_____

_____

_____

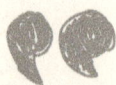

If I cannot do great things, I can do small things in a great way.

Martin Luther King Jr., minister and activist

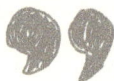

For the last few weeks, you've been taking a moment every so often to think about yourself. You've realised what's great about you, and how you can keep making the most of your circumstances. You've empowered yourself – well done you! Here's to the next fifty-two weeks!

On the following page, note down the activities that were most effective for you and why. How can you continue to incorporate these into your life?

Week _____

New habits I have learned this year:

_____

_____

_____

_____

_____

_____

_____

_____

_____

_____

_____

_____

_____

_____

NOTES

About Trigger Publishing

Trigger is a leading independent altruistic global publisher devoted to opening up conversations about mental health and wellbeing. We share uplifting and inspirational mental health stories, publish advice-driven books by highly qualified clinicians for those in recovery and produce wellbeing books that will help you to live your life with greater meaning and clarity.

Founder Adam Shaw, mental health advocate and philanthropist, established the company with leading psychologist Lauren Callaghan, whilst in recovery from serious mental health issues. Their aim was to publish books which provided advice and support to anyone suffering with mental illness by sharing uplifting and inspiring stories from real life survivors, combined with expert advice on practical recovery techniques.

Since then, Trigger has expanded to produce books on a wide range of topics surrounding mental health and wellness, as well as launching Upside Down, its children's list, which encourages open conversation around mental health from a young age.

We want to help you to not just survive but thrive ... one book at a time.

Find out more about Trigger Publishing by visiting our website: triggerpublishing.com or join us on:
Twitter @TriggerPub
Facebook @TriggerPub
Instagram @TriggerPub

TRIGGER™
The mental health & wellbeing publishe

About Shaw Mind

A proportion of profits from the sale of all Trigger books go to their sister charity, Shaw Mind, also founded by Adam Shaw and Lauren Callaghan. The charity aims to ensure that everyone has access to mental health resources whenever they need them.

You can find out more about the work Shaw Mind do by visiting their website: shawmindfoundation.org or joining them on
Twitter @Shaw_Mind
Facebook @shawmindUK
Instagram @Shaw_Mind

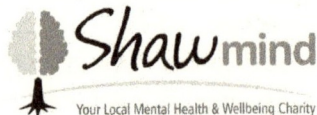

Shawmind

Your Local Mental Health & Wellbeing Charity